The Reproductive System

Kerri O'Donnell

the rosen publishing group's
rosen
central

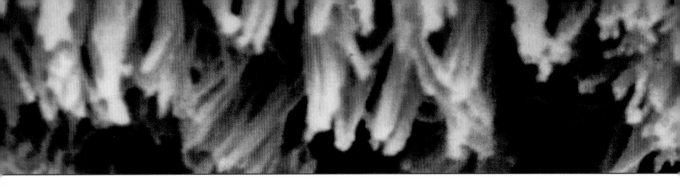

To Catherine, Ken, and Erin for their support and encouragement.

Published in 2001 by The Rosen Publishing Group, Inc.
29 East 21st Street, New York, NY 10010

First Edition

Library of Congress Cataloging-in-Publication Data

O'Donnell, Kerri, 1972–
    The reproductive system / by Kerri O'Donnell—1st ed.
        p. cm. (The insider's guides to the body)
Includes bibliographical references and index.
    ISBN 0-8239-3334-2 (library binding)
1. Human reproduction—Juvenile literature. 2. Reproductive health—Juvenile literature. 3. Generative organs—Juvenile literature. [1. Reproduction. 2. Sex instruction for teenagers.] I. Title. II. Series.
QP251.5 .O366 2000
612.6—dc21
                                                        00-009754

Manufactured in the United States of America

Contents

1 What Is Reproduction, Anyway?

Reproduction. It's a big, stuffy-sounding word that means something quite simple—how having sex makes babies. Before you start blushing and run out of the room in embarrassment, take a deep breath and consider this: Sex is the reason you're here in the first place. And, although it might make you cringe to think about it, sex is how your parents made you.

You may have found yourself thinking about sex lately. After all, you are at an age when all sorts of thoughts and questions may start popping up in your mind. This will happen at the weirdest times—in the middle of a math test, or when you pass that really cute girl or guy in the hallway at school. You might feel like you're the only person in the whole world who has sex on the brain, even if you don't know much about sex at all.

Well, take heart. You're not the only one. As a matter of fact, you're just like everybody else. It's perfectly normal to think about it, to wonder about it, and to talk about it. In fact, maybe you've

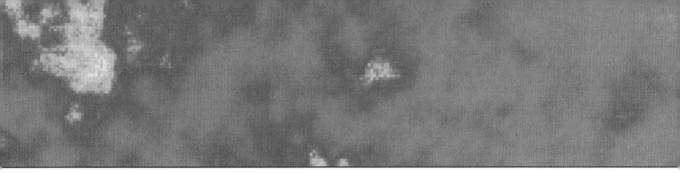

already talked with your parents or with an older brother or sister about sex. Maybe you've been talking about it with your friends. On the other hand, maybe you don't want to talk about it with anyone because you feel too embarrassed.

What you need to remember is that sex is nothing to be embarrassed about. It is a basic human function, and humankind could not continue to exist without it. So it makes sense that you should know what sex is all about, right? The first step is to understand your body, inside and out, and then you can get a handle on how this whole sex/reproduction thing works.

The Amazing Human Body

The human body is an amazing thing. It's capable of everything from running marathons and building skyscrapers to baking cookies. Human beings have discovered cures for illnesses and have invented machines that can take them into outer space. But perhaps the most amazing thing we can do is something that we all kind of take for granted—we can create other living, breathing human beings.

The next time you see a pregnant woman, consider just how incredible it is that people are capable of such a feat. Reproduction might be something you never really thought about, and you might not know exactly how a woman becomes pregnant. Or maybe you think you already know everything there is to know about where babies come from. Either way, there's always more to learn.

The Basics

Human beings, like most animals, reproduce sexually. A human baby is created when a female sex cell and a male sex cell unite. These sex cells are called gametes. Male gametes are called sperm; female gametes are called ova, or eggs. When a sperm and an egg are united, a process called fertilization occurs. A fertilized egg grows into a baby inside a woman's body. This is called pregnancy, and it lasts for approximately nine months.

When fertilization first takes place, the fertilized egg is smaller than the head of a pin. The fertilized egg grows into a group of cells called an embryo. The cells form tissues, and then organs develop. At this point, the embryo is called a fetus. During the rest of the pregnancy, the fetus continues to grow and develop. After about nine months, the fetus is fully developed and can live outside of the mother's body. Pregnancy ends when the woman gives birth to the baby.

HOW OTHER CULTURES VIEW SEX

Cultures around the world look at sex in different ways:

- The Hopi accept their children's sexual curiosity and allow them to masturbate openly.
- The inhabitants of Tepoztlan, Mexico, forbid girls who have had their first menstrual period to talk to boys at all.
- In Indonesia, the Dani people sometimes avoid sexual intercourse for up to six years following childbirth.
- In India, the Chenchu people believe that a child will be born blind if its mother becomes pregnant at night.

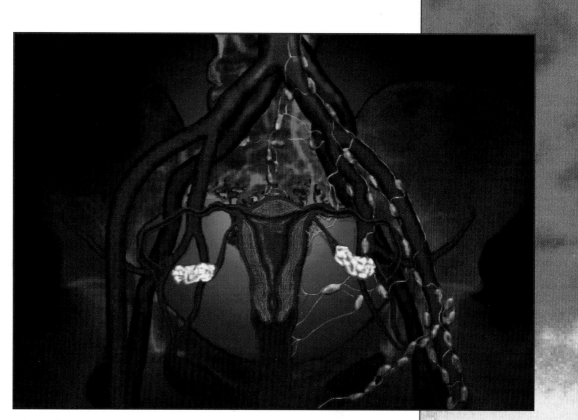

This illustration shows the female reproductive organs: the uterus, vagina, and fallopian tubes.

What Does All This Have to Do with Me?

Plenty. After all, this is how you came into the world. It might seem that reproduction doesn't have much to do with you right now, but someday it might, and it's best to be prepared. Besides, you're at the age when you might be noticing changes in your body, and maybe you're wondering what it all means. Read on, and you'll find out.

2
Puberty Strikes!

Puberty is usually defined as the period in a young person's life when he or she becomes capable of sexual reproduction. There are all kinds of changes that take place before this happens. These changes signal the passage from childhood to adulthood, and mark the beginning of a very exciting time in a person's life—even if it doesn't seem so great while you're living through it!

Puberty can be a confusing time. For one thing, it may seem like your body changes overnight. Your whole body grows (sometimes so quickly that you seem to grow out of a pair of jeans every few weeks). Pimples appear. Your genitals begin to grow and change. Hair starts sprouting up under your arms and around your genitals—places where it doesn't seem like hair should be. Boys might see some stray facial hairs, their voices will begin to get deeper, and they'll have their first (of many) wet dreams. Girls will begin to get their period, or menstruate, and will begin to develop breasts.

It will all feel pretty overwhelming, but you're not the only one having to deal with all of these changes. Everyone—absolutely

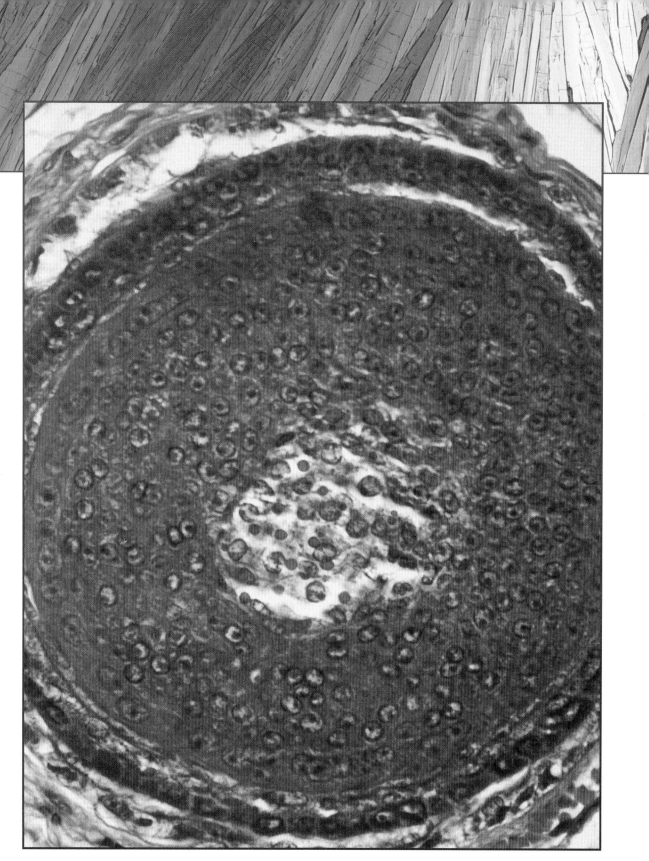

This image shows a cross section of a strand of hair.

everyone—goes through this, and you WILL survive. You just need to understand the reasons behind this seemingly sudden transformation.

It's All in Your Mind

"All in my mind?" you say. "But look at my body! It's going haywire!"

You've got a good point there, but all these changes actually do start in your brain. It all has to do with hormones—chemicals in your body that control everything that happens during puberty.

When puberty begins, a part of the brain called the hypothalamus starts to release large amounts of something called the gonadotropin-releasing hormone. (Try saying that five times fast!) This hormone acts on the brain's pituitary gland. The pituitary gland has the job of releasing secretions that affect most of the body's basic functions. The pituitary gland is stimulated by the gonadotropin-releasing hormone and begins to secrete the gonadotropic hormones. These hormones act on the gonads, or sex glands—the ovaries in females and the testes in males.

The gonads begin to grow and start secreting what are called sex hormones. In males, these sex hormones include testosterone and androsterone, which are called androgens. In females, these sex hormones include progesterone and estrogen, which are called estrogens. Sex hormones regulate the changes that take place during puberty. They are responsible for a person's growth and weight gain. They also tell your body when to stop growing.

In males, androgens make the sex organs grow and develop. They make the voice deepen and cause the growth of facial hair. In females, estrogen makes the sex organs grow and develop. It also makes the hips grow wider and the breasts grow fuller. In females, the estrogen, progesterone, and gonadotropic hormones work together to regulate the menstrual cycle.

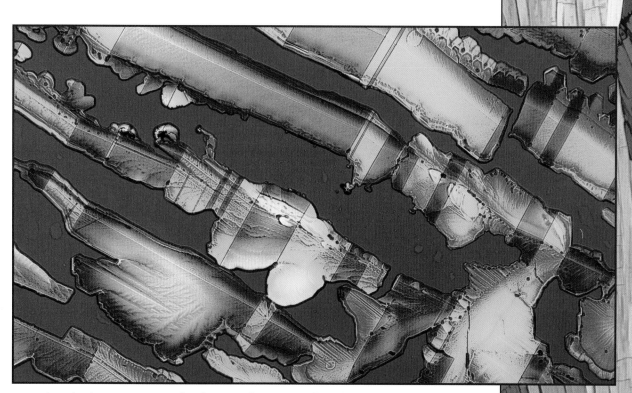

This light micrograph shows the crystals of a type of estrogen, the hormone responsible for female reproduction and the development of secondary sex characteristics.

Now that you know what makes puberty happen, it's time to take a look at how it happens and what it means to you.

Ladies First

Okay, ladies, this section's for you. (Gentlemen, feel free to read along. After all, it can't hurt to know as much as possible about women, can it?)

Typically, girls start puberty anywhere between ages nine and fourteen, the average age being anywhere from ten to twelve years old. Boys go through puberty a bit later. Of course, the age when puberty begins varies, and you shouldn't worry about your body's schedule. You might have felt like you were the only ten-year-old girl in

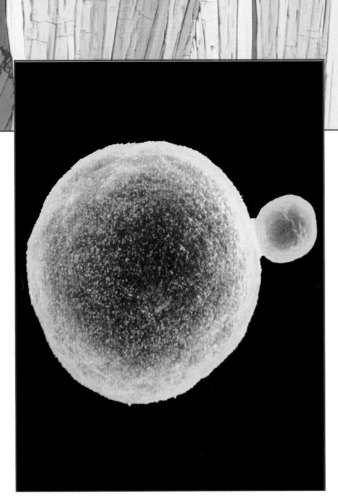

Before ovulation, the human egg is split into the secondary oocyte and the first polar body.

your class to get her period, or you might be the only fifteen-year-old girl in your class still waiting to get it. You might be the only eleven-year-old on your block wearing a bra, or you might look at your flat chest and wonder why your best friend has bigger breasts than you do. Either way, you're perfectly normal. Your body knows when to get everything started. No matter how it feels, you're not the only one going through these tough spots.

The Overview

Once puberty begins, your breasts will get larger and rounder. Your hips will get wider. Pubic hair will start to grow around your vagina, and hair will start to grow under your arms. You might notice some pimples. Your genitals will begin to develop more completely, and you will start to produce mature eggs, or ova (sex cells). This means that it's now possible for you to become pregnant. Yes, you read that right—pregnant. You will also start your menstrual cycle, which is a monthly (and very normal) process. This is such a special event that it deserves its own section.

Say Hello to Your Monthly Visitor

Getting your period for the first time can be scary if you don't know what to expect. You might think you'll never be able to handle this cruel new twist to your life. "I have to deal with this every month?" you might cry in despair. Yes, but you need to realize how important this process is and what it means. Getting your period means that your body is capable of creating a new life.

Hormones

The technical word for getting your period is "menstruation," and it's an important part of a female's reproductive system. Menstruation occurs once a month. Girls have thousands of tiny eggs—or ova—in their ovaries. The ovaries are located near the uterus, the organ in which a baby grows during pregnancy. During menstruation, some eggs begin to mature inside the ovaries. The surrounding cells release an estrogen hormone, which tells the lining of the uterus to thicken with blood and cells so that it can prepare to receive a possible fertilized egg (a pregnancy). The increase in estrogen makes the pituitary gland release a hormone that travels to the ovaries and causes one of the mature eggs to be released. This is called ovulation. The egg moves through the fallopian tube (you have two of these, one for each ovary) on its

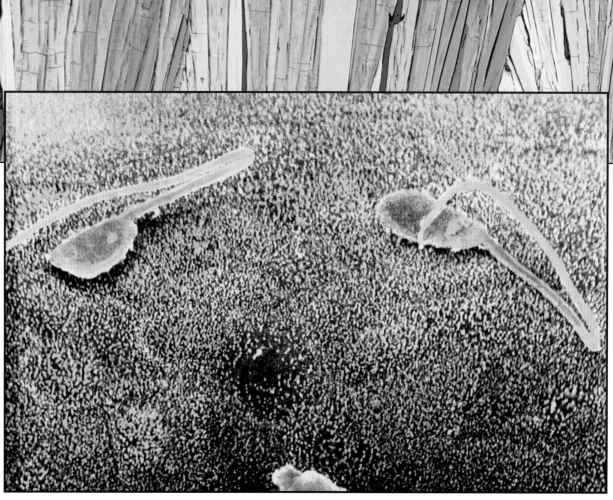

These spermatozoa (shown in yellow), two of about 300 million, did not survive in the uterus and therefore will not fertilize an egg.

way to the uterus. If the egg isn't fertilized and there is no pregnancy, the blood and cells lining the uterus begin to break down and are discharged through the vagina. This process is called menstruation and usually lasts from three to seven days.

Your Turn, Gentlemen

Get ready, guys . . . now it's your turn. (Ladies, sit back and read along!)

Boys start puberty about one year after girls do, the average age being from twelve to fourteen years old. Again, these are just ballpark figures. Don't worry if you're fourteen and don't see any signs of puberty on the horizon—it's coming, you can be sure of it. The same goes for those of you whose voices are changing before anyone else's. Everyone will catch up soon enough.

The Overview

As we've mentioned, once puberty starts, you'll experience changes in your body. You'll grow taller and stronger. Your shoulders will get more broad. Your voice will change, which might be a little embarrassing while it's happening, but will soon sound really cool. You'll start to see pimples here and there. Hair will start growing under your arms and on your face, maybe even on your chest. Pubic hair will start growing around your genitals, which will start to grow and develop. You'll also start to have wet dreams.

Wet WHAT?

Wet dreams are also called nocturnal emissions, and they're absolutely normal. All guys have them. Maybe it has already happened to you—you wake up and realize the bed feels wet. Don't worry, you didn't wet the bed. You've had a wet dream, which means that you've ejaculated in your sleep.

Your reproductive system has reached maturity. Your sex glands (testes) have started to produce testosterone, and that testosterone has begun to produce sperm—the male sex cells that fertilize a woman's egg. If you look at sperm under a microscope, they kind of look like tiny tadpoles, with round heads and little tails. Sperm travel through your body and mix with fluids to form semen. This semen is what comes out of your penis during a wet dream. Wet, sticky spots on your sheets are nothing to worry about.

3
The Female Reproductive System

Now, ladies and gentlemen, it's time to take a closer look at all of the body parts that are involved in the reproductive process. Remember, this is nothing to be squeamish about. The more you know about your body, the more comfortable you'll feel inside your own skin. We'll start with the ladies.

The female reproductive system is a complex system capable of creating another human being. The female body provides a protective place where that human being can grow and develop. In this section, we'll examine the female reproductive organs, both inside and out.

A Look in the Mirror

Let's start with what you can see in the mirror—the external sex organs, or genitals. A female's genitals are sometimes called the vulva, and include the mons veneris, the labia majora, the labia minora, the vestibule, and the clitoris. It might help to use a hand-held mirror to take a closer look at these external organs as they are reviewed.

The mons veneris is the pad of fatty tissue over the pubic bone. It is covered by pubic hair. The labia majora, or outer lips, are the two folds of skin that make up the mons veneris. The labia minora, or inner lips, are the hairless folds of tissue found underneath the outer lips. These inner lips can be seen by separating the outer lips.

The vestibule is found between the inner lips. The opening of the urethra and the vaginal opening are both located in the vestibule, as are two sets

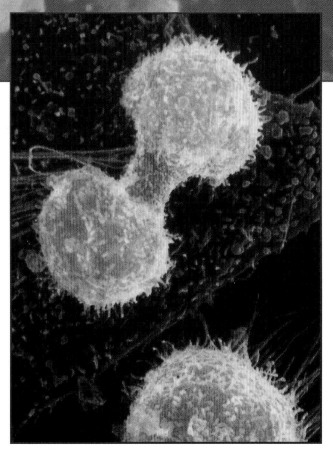

Female egg cell mitosis, or division

of glands. The urethra is a tube that leads from the bladder to the urethral opening in the vestibule. This opening is where urine leaves the body. The vaginal opening is located just beneath the urethral opening, and is the gateway to your internal reproductive organs. It is sometimes partially covered by a very thin layer of skin called the hymen. Outside of the vaginal opening are two sets of Bartholin's glands. When a woman is sexually excited, these glands release a bit of fluid.

The clitoris is located where the labia minora join, just above the vestibule. It is a small organ that contains many nerve endings and is very sensitive to the touch.

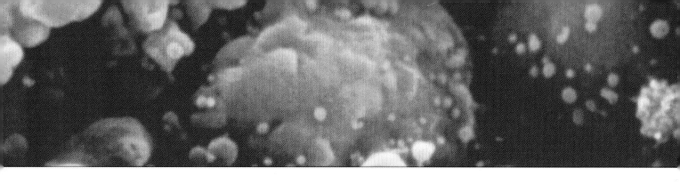

A Look Inside

Now let's take a look at what you can't see in the mirror. The reproductive organs found inside your body consist of the vagina, the uterus (which includes the cervix), the fallopian tubes, and the ovaries.

The vagina is a muscular, tube-shaped organ that leads to the inside of your body. It is about three to five inches long. It can expand in shape and size to fit a male's penis during sexual intercourse, or to serve as the birth passage for a baby. During your period, your menstrual blood exits your body through the vagina.

The uterus, or womb, is a thick, hollow organ shaped like an upside-down pear. It is about the size of your fist, about three inches long and two inches wide, and is made of strong muscle that can expand and stretch to hold a baby. Its job is to receive a fertilized egg and nourish and protect the embryo until childbirth. Each

The uterus, or womb, is a hollow organ made of strong muscle that can expand to hold a fetus. It is connected to the ovaries by the fallopian tubes.

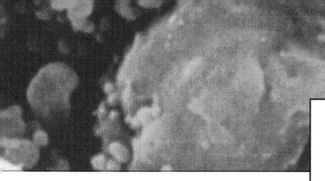

month, the lining of the uterus builds up to provide nourishment to a fertilized egg. If there is no fertilized egg, this lining is shed during menstruation.

The lower third of the uterus is called the cervix. It is narrow and tube-shaped, and is only about one inch in diameter. The cervix is located at the end of the vagina.

Your two fallopian tubes are each about four inches long and extend from either side of your uterus. The ends of the fallopian tubes are funnel-shaped and lined with fimbriae, moving, fingerlike projections that draw an egg into the tube from the ovary.

The ovaries are about the size and shape of almonds and are found near the ends of the fallopian tubes on either side of the uterus. Ovaries produce eggs, or ova, and estrogen and progesterone.

DID YOU KNOW?

● Mons veneris is Latin for "mound of Venus"—Venus was the Roman goddess of beauty.

● A female's clitoris has just as many nerve endings as a male's penis has, even though the clitoris is very small in comparison.

● By about the age of thirty-five, a woman will have only about 30,000 eggs left—about 370,000 fewer than she was born with!

● A woman will ovulate about 400 eggs during her lifetime.

4
The Male Reproductive System

The male reproductive system is just as complex as the female reproductive system. A male's reproductive organs must deliver sperm to the egg of the female in order for fertilization to occur. In this section, we'll take a look at the male reproductive organs and discuss their various functions.

First Things First

Guys, now it's your turn to look in the mirror. What you see are your external reproductive organs—your genitals—the penis and scrotum.

The penis is a cylindrical organ that males use to urinate. The penis also becomes longer and stiffer when a male experiences an erection. The head of the penis is called the glans. In the middle of the glans is the urethral opening, where urine leaves the body. The glans has many nerve endings and is sensitive to the touch. The foreskin is a loose piece of skin that covers the glans. Males who were circumcised as babies have less foreskin. The shaft of the penis extends from the glans to where the penis connects with the body. Loose skin covers the shaft so that it can get bigger during an erection.

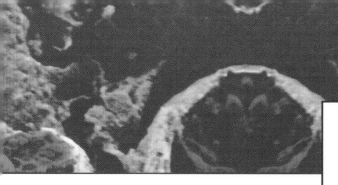

The scrotum is a loose pouch of skin located behind the penis. The skin of the scrotum is darker than the rest of the body's skin and will eventually have a light covering of hair. The scrotum holds the testes, or testicles—the internal male sex glands that produce sperm and testosterone. The scrotum's location outside of the body keeps the testes a few degrees cooler than normal body temperature. The testes need this cooler temperature to produce sperm.

Beneath the Surface

You can't see them, but the male's internal reproductive organs are fascinating structures, and they all have important jobs to do. These organs include the testes, the epididymis, the vas deferens, the seminal vesicles, the prostate gland, and the Cowper's glands.

The two testes are oval-shaped sex glands found inside the scrotum. In an adult male, they are about two inches long and one inch wide. The testes produce testosterone and sperm. Inside the testes are tiny, coiled, tubelike structures called seminiferous tubules. This is where sperm are produced.

Sperm are stored and mature inside the epididymis. The epididymis is a tightly coiled tube located on the surface of each testicle. Sperm

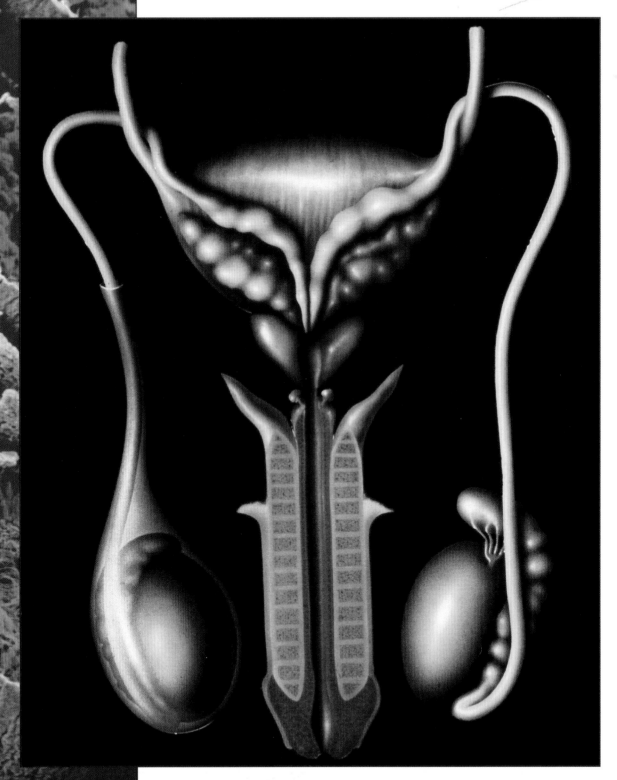

The male reproductive system includes the penis and the oval-shaped testes, in which sperm are produced.

travel from the epididymis through a small tube called the vas deferens. The vas deferens joins with the duct from the seminal vesicle to become the ejaculatory duct.

The seminal vesicles are shaped like small pouches. When a male reaches the peak of excitement during sexual intercourse—or during masturbation (self-stimulation)—he ejaculates. The seminal vesicles release fluid into the ejaculatory ducts, which then mixes with sperm from the vas deferens. The fluid from the seminal vesicles contains a sugar called fructose, which gives the sperm energy to move.

DID YOU KNOW?

- From end to end, a male's epididymis is about twenty feet long!
- If you were to uncoil a male's seminiferous tubules, they would be several thousand feet long
- It takes about seventy-four days for a man to produce new sperm. Each day, 200 million sperm reach maturity after going through this seventy-four-day cycle.

The prostate gland is found below the bladder, just behind the penis and urethra. It is doughnut-shaped and surrounds the urethra. The prostate gland connects the ejaculatory ducts and the urethra. During ejaculation, fluid from the prostate gland mixes with fluid from the ejaculatory ducts to make a fluid called semen. Semen is what comes out of a male's penis when he ejaculates.

The Cowper's glands are found on either side of the urethra, below the prostate gland. When a man is sexually excited, a bit of fluid from these glands is secreted into the urethra. This clear, sticky fluid can sometimes be seen on the tip of the penis right before ejaculation.

5
The Truth About Pregnancy

Now you all know what you've got. Let's take a look at the reproductive process so you can see how the male and female reproductive organs work together to form a new life.

Fertilization

Pregnancy begins when a male's sperm fertilizes a female's egg—also called conception. This usually happens during sexual intercourse. Sexual intercourse is what happens when a male's erect penis is inserted into the female's vagina. The friction caused by the movement of the penis in and out of the vagina stimulates the sex organs. When this sexual stimulation reaches its peak in the male, he has what is called an orgasm and ejaculates. During ejaculation, the male's semen is deposited in the female's vagina.

The semen contains millions of sperm. When a male ejaculates inside the female's vagina, these sperm travel (swim, really) through the cervix into the female's uterus, then make their way

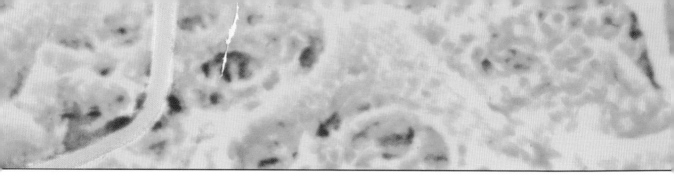

into the fallopian tubes. It's a tough journey for the sperm, and most die in the process. Just a few thousand sperm successfully reach each fallopian tube.

This is where the female's menstrual cycle comes into play. You'll remember from chapter 2 that each month, a mature egg is released from one of the female's ovaries into one of the fallopian tubes. If sperm comes into contact with the egg as it travels through the fallopian tube on its way to the uterus, fertilization can occur.

The Battle of the Sperm

Sperm are tiny, so tiny that you need a microscope to even see them. When a man ejaculates, the semen that is released (usually less than a teaspoonful) contains millions of sperm. Typically, only one sperm fertilizes an egg, although it's likely that several hundred sperm have reached the egg. That's a lot of competition—not only to get to the egg first, but to pass through the egg's protective covering in order to fertilize it.

Some sperm can reach the fallopian tubes in just minutes, but other sperm take hours to make the trip. Once they are inside the fallopian tubes, sperm can live for forty-eight to seventy-two hours. After a female ovulates, it takes the egg about seventy-two hours to travel through the fallopian tube. If any sperm meet up with the egg as the egg makes its way down one of the fallopian tubes on its way to the uterus, fertilization can result.

Breaking and Entering

The egg is covered with two layers of cells a sperm must get through in order to fertilize the egg. Inside the rounded head of the sperm—called the acrosome—are chemicals that dig a hole in the egg's protective covering. Many sperm may start to penetrate the egg's layers, but only one sperm can usually get inside to fertilize the egg. When this lucky sperm makes it inside the egg, the egg lets off chemicals that make it impossible for other sperm to enter.

When the sperm's chromosomes join with the egg's chromosomes, fertilization is complete. Chromosomes are tiny structures shaped like rods that are found in the nucleus, or center, of both male and female sex cells. Chromosomes contain genes, which are passed down from generation to generation and are responsible for each individual's unique traits.

The Embryo

The fertilized egg, which is smaller than a grain of sand, is called a zygote. It contains forty-six chromosomes, twenty-three from the egg and twenty-three from the sperm. Before it even reaches the uterus, the zygote undergoes several changes. After fertilization, the zygote moves through the fallopian tube toward the uterus. The zygote begins to divide—one cell becomes two cells, two become four, four become eight, and so on. The zygote is now called an embryo.

The embryo reaches the uterus about three days after fertilization and implants itself in the uterine lining. The embryo begins to secrete a hormone called human chorionic gonadotropin (hCG). This hormone stops the menstrual cycle, and the pregnant female no longer gets her period.

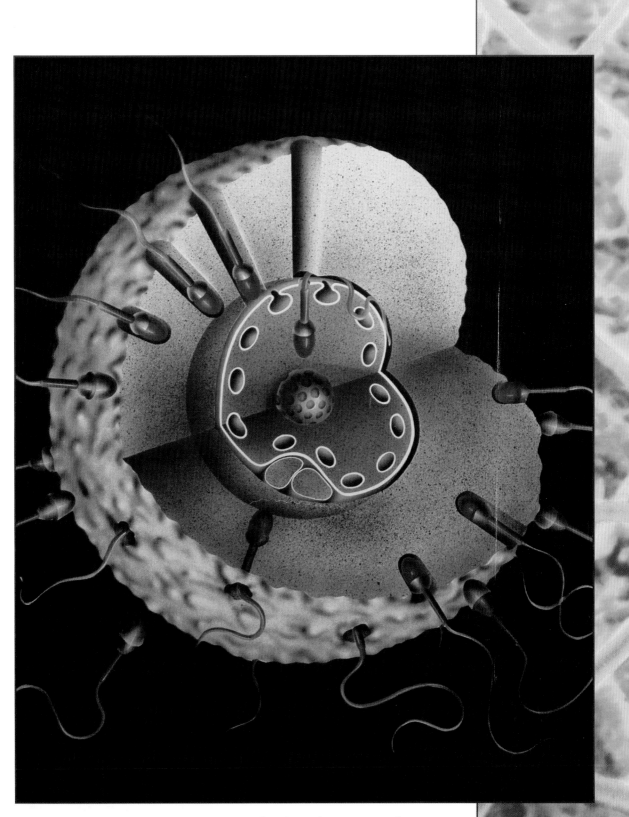

A sperm must penetrate the egg to fertilize the egg. Only one sperm is usually able to do this. When the sperm's chromosomes join with the egg's chromosomes, fertilization is complete.

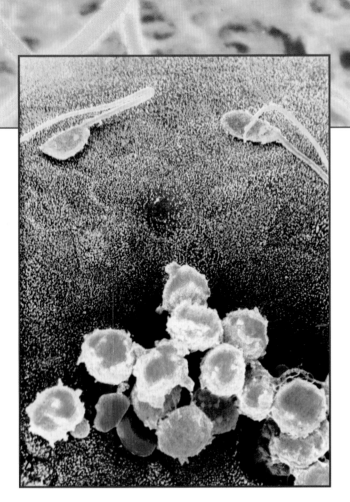

Once inside the fallopian tubes, sperm can live anywhere from two to three days.

SIGNS OF PREGNANCY

- A missed or abnormally light period
- Sore, tender breasts
- Increased fatigue
- Increased nausea
- Change in appetite
- More frequent urination

From Embryo to Fetus

Within the first two weeks of pregnancy, structures that will help the embryo grow begin to form in the uterus. One of these structures is a disk-shaped organ called the placenta. The placenta removes the embryo's waste materials and supplies it with oxygen and food. It also makes hormones that control the embryo's development.

All of the embryo's major organs start to form between the third and the eighth week of pregnancy. The embryo is about an inch long and weighs about half an ounce by the end of the second month. At around the ninth week, the baby's body begins to grow and its organs begin to develop. From this point until childbirth, the baby is called a fetus. During the first three months of the fetus

The fetus experiences dramatic increases in size and weight, especially during the second and third trimesters of pregnancy.

stage, the length of the fetus increases dramatically, growing as much as two inches each month. During the last months of pregnancy, the weight of the fetus greatly increases as well.

Stages of Fetal Growth

Pregnancy is divided into three equal parts, which are called trimesters. Each trimester lasts for three months. After the second trimester, the fetus is nearly five times longer and weighs about thirty times as much. Just before childbirth, the fetus is about twenty inches long and weighs (on average) around seven pounds.

The Baby Makes an Entrance

Pregnancy usually lasts for about forty weeks (roughly nine months). When it's time for the child to be born, the woman goes into labor. During labor, the child is pushed out of the uterus. The process of labor is divided into three stages.

During the first stage, a woman experiences labor pains—discomfort caused by muscles in the uterus as they tense up and then relax. Then the cervix opens, or dilates. When the cervix has fully dilated—about four inches in diameter—the second stage begins. Muscle contractions in the uterus and abdomen begin to push the baby through the cervix, and then through the vagina.

The third stage begins once the baby is born. It ends when the placenta—the organ that has been nourishing the baby inside the womb—is pushed out of the uterus and vagina.

Infertility

When a couple can't produce children through sexual intercourse, this is called infertility. Sometimes the man has a problem with his reproductive system, which affects the sperm in his semen. Sometimes the woman has a problem with her reproductive system, such as a blockage of her fallopian tubes, which carry eggs from the ovaries to the uterus. Fortunately, there are alternatives.

MEDICAL MIRACLES FOR INFERTILITY PATIENTS

- Artificial insemination is a procedure in which semen is injected into a woman's uterus. Sometimes the male's semen is "washed" to remove unhealthy sperm, antibodies, and seminal fluid that could be rejected by the female's uterus. At the doctor's office, the healthy sperm are placed directly inside the uterus. If the male's sperm aren't capable of fertilization, donor sperm may be used.

- Laser surgery can often permanently cure some kinds of infertility, especially when infertility is caused by a blockage in the fallopian tubes. In this procedure, an intense beam of light is aimed at the blockage to remove it.

- In a process called in vitro fertilization, eggs are removed from the female and fertilized by the male's sperm with microscopic instruments. This takes place in a laboratory. During an office visit, the fertilized eggs are then implanted into the female's uterus. Donor eggs can be used if the female's eggs are damaged.

6

Play It Safe

Your body is growing, your genitals are maturing, your hormones are going wild, and you have sex on the brain. Someday, you might be asking yourself if you're ready for a sexual relationship. This is a very personal issue—no one knows the answer but you. If you don't know for sure if you're ready, then you're not, no matter what anyone else might try to tell you. But if and when you do decide that you're ready, it's very important to know about birth control. Pregnancy is one of the biggest decisions you'll ever make in your life, and it should be just that—a decision. If you have sex without birth control, the decision is no longer yours to make. Having unprotected sexual intercourse just one time—even if it's your very first time—can result in pregnancy.

The Benefits of Birth Control

Many people think that using birth control products (also called contraceptives) is too much trouble, and that it ruins the "mood." The simple fact is that the few moments it takes to use contraceptives can

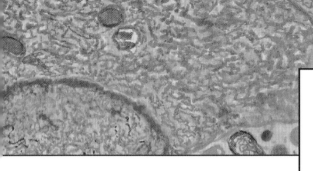

prevent an unwanted pregnancy. Certain contraceptives can also protect you from sexually transmitted diseases (STDs) like herpes, chlamydia, and AIDS. To be effective (that is, to keep the reproductive system from reproducing), contra-

ceptives must be used every single time a person has sexual intercourse. Young women should see a gynecologist—a doctor who specializes in the female body and reproductive system—who will help determine what form of birth control is best for each individual.

Abstinence, the Rhythm Method, and Withdrawal

Abstinence means that a person does not have sexual intercourse at all. It is the only 100 percent effective method of birth control. If you don't have sexual intercourse, you can't get pregnant or get someone else pregnant.

Using the rhythm method means that a man and woman do not have sex during the time of the month when the woman is ovulating. This isn't an effective method of birth control because sperm can live inside the vagina for several days. Therefore, a woman should not have sex for a few days before and five days after she

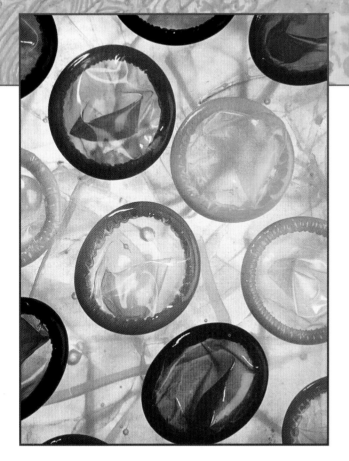

Because a condom prevents the exchange of body fluids, it is very effective in protecting against both pregnancy and STDs.

ovulates. However, keep in mind that it can be difficult to accurately predict the exact moment of ovulation. This method also doesn't protect against STDs.

When a man practices withdrawal, he takes his penis out of the woman's vagina before he ejaculates. This method is ineffective because semen can leak out of the penis before ejaculation. This method doesn't protect you from STDs either.

The Pill

The pill is a very reliable method of birth control, and it's easy to use. The female simply takes one pill each day. The pill contains hormones that simulate pregnancy, so the ovaries don't release any new eggs. The pill can be prescribed by a gynecologist and comes in packages that contain a monthly supply. If used alone as a method of birth control, the pill does not protect against STDs.

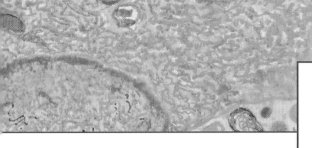

Condoms, Diaphragms, and Cervical Caps

A condom is a sheath of rubber that fits over a male's erect penis. It is put on before sexual intercourse takes place and acts as a barrier between the male's sperm and the female's vagina. Because a condom prevents the exchange of body fluids, it's very effective in protecting against both pregnancy and STDs. Condoms can be bought at most drugstores and grocery stores.

A diaphragm looks like a little rubber bowl. To use the diaphragm correctly, it should be filled with spermicide, a chemical that kills sperm, and put into the vagina so that it covers the cervical opening. The diaphragm's job is to stop sperm from getting inside the uterus. If any sperm manage to get around the diaphragm, the spermicide kills them. Women can be fitted by a gynecologist to ensure that the diaphragm is the proper size for her body. The diaphragm is an effective method of birth control when used properly.

A cervical cap is really just a miniature version of a diaphragm. Like a diaphragm, it's made of rubber and fits over the opening of the cervix. A gynecologist can ensure the proper fit.

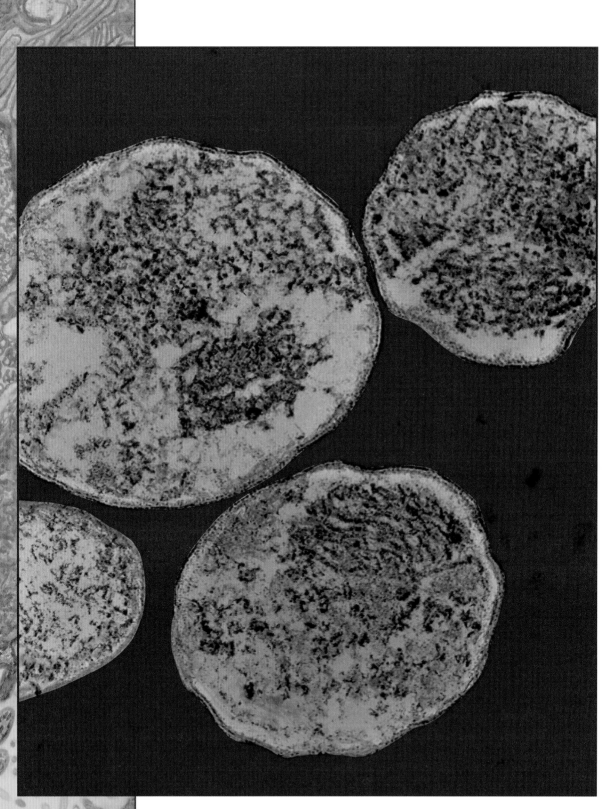

These bacteria (shown magnified 74,000x) cause chlamydia, a sexually transmitted disease.

More Birth Control Information

- Spermicides are designed to be used with condoms, diaphragms, and cervical caps in order to make these forms of birth control more effective. Spermicides may also help to prevent some STDs. However, spermicides are very ineffective against pregnancy when used alone.

- The female condom is like a male condom but larger. It has an inner rim that fits over the cervix and an outer rim that fits over the labia.

- Norplant is a set of small capsules that are implanted in a woman's arm. They slowly dissolve, releasing synthetic hormones that halt ovulation and prevent pregnancy. Norplant works for several years at a time.

- Depo-Provera is an injection of synthetic hormones given to women that stops ovulation and prevents pregnancy. It is effective for up to three months.

All in Good Time

Sex, babies, birth control . . . getting older is complicated stuff! However, now that you know how your reproductive system works, you should feel better equipped to deal with the process of growing up.

Glossary

acrosome   Structure found in the head of sperm that contains chemicals that eat through an egg's protective layers

androgens   Male hormones that are responsible for the development of male sexual characteristics.

androsterone   Male hormone.

Bartholin's glands   Small glands found on either side of the vaginal opening that secrete fluid.

cervix   Narrow lower third of the uterus that is connected to the vagina.

chlamydia   Infection of the genitals caused by bacteria.

chromosome   Rodlike structure in the nucleus of a cell that contains hereditary information.

clitoris   Small, sensitive organ found at the top of the vestibule in females.

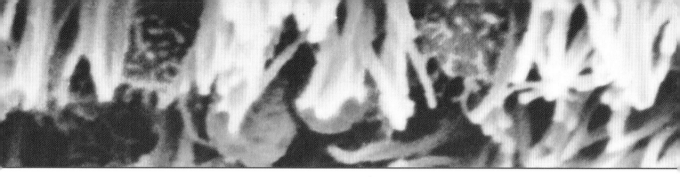

contraceptive Drug or device used during sex to prevent pregnancy.

Cowper's glands Two glands found beneath the prostate gland on either side of a male's urethra.

ejaculation Sudden release of semen through the penis.

embryo Unborn child during the first eight weeks of development.

epididymis Tightly coiled structure found on the back surface of each testicle.

erection Stiffening and lengthening of the penis.

estrogen Hormone that is responsible for the development of female sexual characteristics.

fallopian tube Tube that carries an egg from the ovary to the uterus. It also carries the sperm from the uterus toward the ovary.

fertilization Joining of the male sperm and the female egg.

fetus Unborn child from about the eighth week of development until childbirth.

gamete Mature female or male sex cell; the egg or the sperm.

gonad Sex gland in a male or female; the testis in the male and the ovary in the female.

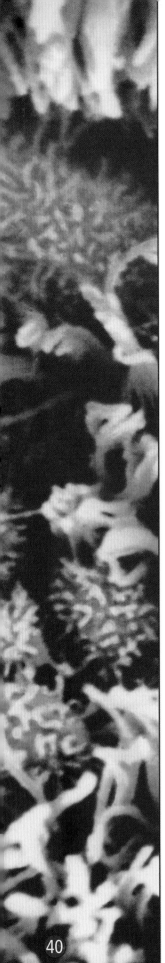

gonadotropin-releasing hormone   Hormone that acts upon the pituitary gland, causing it to release hormones that affect the gonads.

gynecologist   Doctor who specializes in the female body and reproductive system.

human chorionic gonadotropin   Hormone produced by the embryo and fetus.

hymen   Thin piece of skin that sometimes covers the vaginal opening.

hypothalamus   Part of the brain that secretes hormones that regulate various body processes.

labia majora   Outer lips of the vagina.

labia minora   Inner lips of the vagina.

menstruation   Monthly discharge of blood from the lining of the uterus.

mons veneris   Fatty, hair-covered pad of tissue that covers the female's pubic bone.

nocturnal emission   Ejaculation the male has during sleep. Also called a wet dream.

orgasm   Series of pleasurable muscle contractions that occurs at the peak of sexual excitement.

ovary   One of a pair of female sex glands in which hormones and female sex cells, or ova, are produced.

pituitary gland   Gland at the base of the brain that secretes hormones that regulate many body processes.

placenta   Organ that connects a fetus to the mother's uterus. It provides the fetus with oxygen and food, and removes fetal waste.

progesterone   Female hormone secreted by the ovaries.

prostate gland   Gland that surrounds the urethra in the male. It secretes a fluid that helps sperm move.

scrotum   Loose pouch of skin that holds the testes.

semen   Sticky, grayish white fluid that is expelled from the male's urethra during ejaculation.

seminal vesicle   One of two glands in the male that secretes a fluid that is found in semen.

seminiferous tubules   Tiny, tightly coiled tubes in the testes that produce sperm.

testis   One of a pair of male sex glands that produces sperm and testosterone. Also called a testicle.

testosterone   Hormone made by the testes that plays a large role in male sexual development and functioning.

urethra   Duct through which urine leaves the bladder and exits the body.

uterus   Female organ in which an unborn child is contained and nourished until birth. Also called the womb.

vas deferens   Small tube that carries sperm from the epididymis to the ejaculatory duct.

vestibule   Area between the labia minora.

zygote   Fertilized egg.

For More Information

In the United States

American Social Health Association
P. O. Box 13827
Research Triangle Park, NC 27709
(919) 361-8400
Web site: http://www.ashastd.org

America's Crisis Pregnancy Helpline
2121 Valley View Lane
Dallas, TX 75234
(888) 4-OPTIONS (467-8466)
Web site: http://thehelpline.org

Henry J. Kaiser Family Foundation
2400 Sand Hill Road

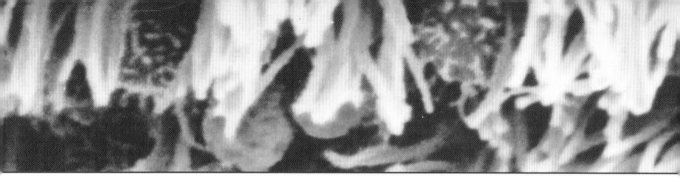

Menlo Park, CA 94025
(650) 854-9400
Web site: http://www.kff.org

National Campaign to Prevent Teen Pregnancy
1776 Massachusetts Avenue NW, Suite 200
Washington, DC 20036
(202) 478-8500
Web site: http://www.teenpregnancy.org

National Women's Health Network
514 10th Street NW, Suite 400
Washington, DC 20004
(202) 347-1140

Planned Parenthood Federation of America
810 Seventh Avenue
New York, NY 10019
(800) 230-7526
Web site: http://www.plannedparenthood.org

Sex Information and Education Council of the United States (SIECUS)
130 West 42nd Street
New York, NY 10036
(212) 819-9770
Web site: http://www.siecus.org

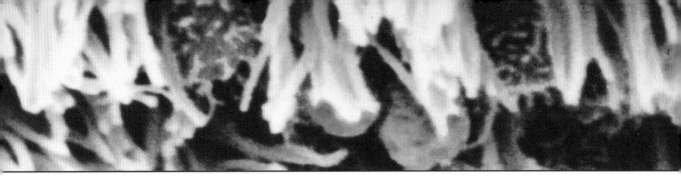

In Canada

Planned Parenthood Federation of Canada
1 Nicholas Street, Suite 430
Ottawa, ON K1N 7B7
Web site: http://www.ppfc.ca

Sex Information and Education Council of Canada (SIECCAN)
850 Coxwell Avenue
Toronto, ON M4C 5R1
(416) 466-5304
Web site: http://www.sieccan.org

Web Sites

Dr. Paula
http://www.drpaula.com

Kids Health
http://www.kidshealth.org

Sex Etc.—A Web Site by Teens for Teens
http://www.sxetc.org

For Further Reading

Golliher, Catherine. *Puberty and Reproduction.* Santa Cruz, CA: ETR Associates, 1996.

Harris, Robie H. *It's Perfectly Normal: Changing Bodies, Growing Up, Sex, and Sexual Health.* Cambridge, MA: Candlewick Press, 1994.

Kelly, Bill. *You Ought to Know: A Guy's Guide to Sex.* New York: Rosen Publishing Group, 2000.

Madaras, Lynda, and Area Madaras. *My Body, My Self for Girls.* New York: Newmarket Press, 1993.

Martin, Karin A. *Puberty, Sexuality, and the Self: Boys and Girls at Adolescence.* New York: Routledge, 1996.

Mucciolo, Gary. *Everything You Need to Know About Birth Control.* New York: Rosen Publishing Group, 1998.

Shaw, Victoria F. *Body Talk: A Girl's Guide to What's Happening to Your Body.* New York: Rosen Publishing Group, 1999.

Westheimer, Ruth K. *Dr. Ruth Talks to Kids: Where You Came from, How Your Body Changes, and What Sex Is All About*. Madison, WI: Demco Media, Limited, 1998.

Index

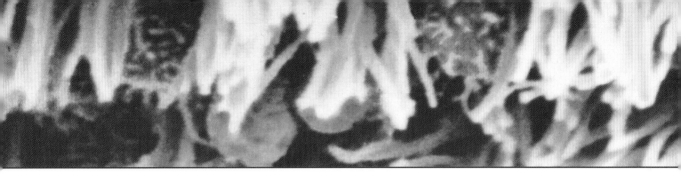

H
hormones, 10, 26, 28, 32, 34, 37
hymen, 17

I
infertility, 30–31, 35
in vitro fertilization, 31

L
labia, 16, 17, 37

M
masturbation, 6, 23
menstruation, 6, 8, 10, 12, 13–14, 18–19, 25, 26, 28
mons veneris, 16, 17, 19

N
Norplant, 37

O
ovaries, 10, 13, 18, 19, 25, 30, 34
ovulation, 13, 19, 25, 33–34, 37

P
penis, 15, 18, 19, 20, 21, 23, 24, 34, 35
pill, birth control, 34
pimples, 8, 12, 15
pituitary gland, 10, 13
placenta, 28, 30
pregnancy, 5, 6, 12, 13, 14, 24–31, 32, 33, 34, 35, 37
progesterone, 10, 19
prostate gland, 21, 23
puberty, 8–15
    in boys, 8, 10, 14–15
    in girls, 8, 10, 11–14

R
reproductive system,
    female, 16–19
    male, 20–23
rhythm method, 33–34

S
semen, 15, 23, 24, 25, 30, 31, 34
seminal vesicles, 21, 23
sexual intercourse, 4–5, 6, 18, 23, 24, 25, 30, 32, 33, 35, 37
sexually transmitted diseases (STDs), 33, 34, 35, 37
sperm, 6, 15, 20, 21, 23, 24–25, 26, 30, 31, 34, 35
spermicide, 35, 37

T
testes, 10, 15, 21, 23
testosterone, 10, 15, 21

U
urethra, 17, 20, 23
uterus, 13, 14, 18, 19, 24, 25, 26, 28, 30, 31, 35

V
vagina, 12, 14, 17, 18, 19, 24, 30, 34, 35
vas deferens, 21, 23
vulva, 16

W
wet dreams, 8, 15
withdrawal, 33, 34

Z
zygote, 26

Credits

About the Author

Kerri O'Donnell received a B.A. in journalism from New York University. She is a writer and editor currently living in Buffalo, New York.

Photo Credits

P. 7 © Photo Researchers, Inc.; p. 9 © 1991 Keith/Custom Medical Stock Photo; p. 11 © 1998 SPL/Custom Medical Stock Photo; pp.12, 14, 28 © Prof. P. Motta/Dept. of Anatomy/University "La Sapienza," Rome/Science Photo Library; p. 17 © SPL/Custom Medical Stock Photo; pp. 18, 29 © Life ART; p. 22 © Francis Leroy, Biocosmos/Science Photo Library; p. 27 © Francis Leroy, Biocosmos/Science Photo Library; p. 34 © Phillip Hayson/Photo Researchers, Inc; p. 36 © Dr. Kari Lounatmaa/Science Photo Library.

Cover, front matter and back matter © Dr. Yorgos Nikas/Science Photo Library: sperm in a fallopian tube.
Ch. 1 © Richard G. Rawlins, Ph.D./Custom Medical Stock Photo: sperm entering an egg.
Ch. 2 © Alfred Pasieka/Science Photo Library: female sex hormone magnified 20x.
Ch. 3 © 1992 SPL/Custom Medical Stock Photo: primordial female egg cell.
Ch. 4 © CNRI/Science Photo Library: seminiferous tubules magnified 72x.
Ch. 5 © Dr. Yorgos Nikas/Science Photo Library: sperm fertilizing an egg, magnified 2,600x.
Ch. 6 © Dr. R. Dourmashkin/Science Photo Library: chlamydial infection of the fallopian tube.

Series Design and Layout

Cindy Williamson